User Guide

for

Health Assessment Online for
Physical Examination and Health Assessment

Fourth Edition

PREPARED BY

Thom Mansen, PhD, RN
Associate Professor of Nursing
College of Nursing
The University of Utah
Salt Lake City, Utah

Kris Robinson, PhD, FNP, RN
Professor of Nursing
Department of Nursing
Idaho State University
Pocatello, Idaho

CONTRIBUTOR

Rae W. Langford, EdD, RN
Private Practice
Rehabilitation Nurse Consultant
Legal Nurse Consultant
Research and Statistics Consultant
Houston, Texas

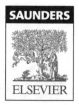

SAUNDERS

ELSEVIER

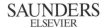

SAUNDERS
ELSEVIER

The Curtis Center
Independence Square West
Philadelphia, Pennsylvania 19106-3399

HEALTH ASSESSMENT ONLINE FOR
PHYSICAL EXAMINATION AND
HEALTH ASSESSMENT
Fourth Edition
Copyright © 2003, Elsevier (USA). All rights reserved.

NOTICE

Health care is an ever-changing field. Standard safety precautions
must be followed, but as new research and clinical experience
broaden our knowledge, changes in treatment and drug therapy may
become necessary or appropriate. Readers are advised to check the
most current product information provided by the manufacturer of
each drug to be administered to verify the recommended dose, the
method and duration of administration, and contraindications. It is
the responsibility of the licensed prescriber, relying on experience
and knowledge of the patient, to determine dosages and the best
treatment for each individual patient. Neither the publisher nor the
editor assumes any liability for any injury and/or damage to persons
or property arising from this publication.

ISBN-13: 978-0-7216-9364-4
ISBN-10: 0-7216-9364-4

Evolve® is a registered trademark of Elsevier Inc. in the United States and/or other jurisdictions.

Vice President and Publishing Director: Sally Schrefer
Executive Editor: Robin Carter
Developmental Editor: Lauren Borstell
Publishing Services Manager: Gayle May
Multimedia Producer: Tyson Sturgeon
Online Development Team: Brent Bailey, Ange Hemmer, Shephali Graf

Printed in the United States of America

Last digit is the print number: 9 8 7

Getting Started

If your course is being led by an instructor:

1. System

Your instructor will provide information about the system on which your course is being hosted. Evolve® courses can be run on a variety of systems and your instructor will decide which one is right for this course.

2. Username & Password

Your instructor will also provide you with the username and password needed to access the system where this course is located.

3. Login Instructions

If your instructor's course is being hosted on the Evolve Learning System, please go to page 12 for instructions about how to log in. If your course is on a different system, your instructor will provide information about how to log in.

4. Access Code

The first time you access this course, you will need the access code located inside the front cover of this User Guide, regardless of which system is hosting the course. When you are prompted, enter the code exactly as it appears in this guide.

If you plan to take the course on your own:

(**Note:** By taking the course independently, you will not have any instructor to help you with the course. You will have 12 months from the date you are enrolled to complete the course.)

1. System

All independent learners are enrolled in a course hosted on the Evolve Learning System.

2. Self-Enrollment

Please go to page 12 for the instructions about how to self-enroll in the course.

3. Username & Password

If you don't have an existing Evolve account, you will be able to create one during the self-enrollment process.

4. Login Instructions

Please go to page 12 for instructions about how to log in to the Evolve Learning System.

5. Access Code

The first time you access this course, you will need the access code located inside the front cover of this User Guide. When you are prompted, enter the code **exactly** as it appears in this guide.

WHAT IS AN ONLINE LEARNING LIBRARY?

An online learning library is a collection of web-based content and interactive tools designed to help you understand and apply even the most complex topics in your studies. The material focuses on a single academic subject and is designed to be used as either a reference library for learning or to complement your instructor's class. Combining proven learning strategies with the best in web technology, this resource strengthens your knowledge and expands your classroom and independent learning experiences. Its features include:

- Multimedia-rich explanation of key concepts, using all the advantages of the web (animations, video, audio, images, interactive exercises, communication tools, hyperlinks, and more) to deepen your learning beyond the capabilities of most study aids.
- Point-and-click tools that help you interact with the chapter material, expanding and deepening the learning process.
- Tools that help you manage your time, check your progress, prepare for exams, organize your notes, and more.
- Dynamic feedback on your answers to quiz questions that provides immediate reinforcement of your learning and guidance for further study.
- Tools that allow you to customize the online learning resource materials to fit your study habits.

WHAT IS HEALTH ASSESSMENT ONLINE?

Health Assessment Online is a rich library of animations, interactive exercises, video clips, audio clips, quizzes, images, and more. Review them once, review them twice, review them whenever you want. Some of the materials, such as animations and video clips, may be linked to for use in your projects or assignments. Resources such as the images may be downloaded for your convenience. Remember that whenever you use these materials outside of this program, you must provide the appropriate references.

The Details of Health Assessment Online

To access the components of Health Assessment Online, navigate to the **Course Documents** area of the course (Note: The location of the Course Documents area will vary depending on the system [Blackboard, WebCT, etc.] the course is hosted on.) Inside this area of the course will be all of the contents for each chapter of this course. You will also find the glossary and the laboratory and diagnostic tests.

Chapter Folders

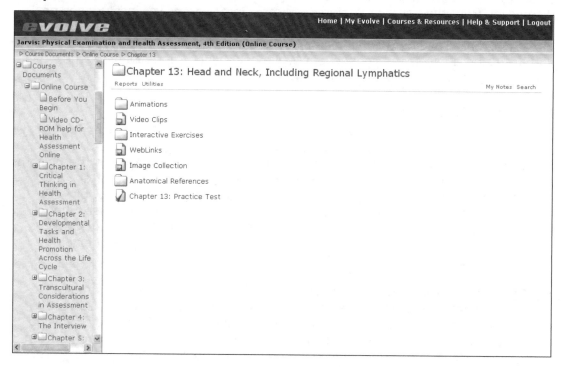

Each **Chapter Folder** contains a variety of educational tools, such as animations, video clips, interactive exercises, WebLinks, images, anatomical references, and practice tests. Chapters 18 and 19 also include audio clips. When you click on any given chapter, links to each of the tools will appear. Click on the link to access the content you wish to use.

Animations

Sixty-five animations bring important anatomical and physiological concepts to life. When you click on the **Animations** link inside the **Chapter Folder**, a list of links to specific animations will appear. Click on the animation of your choice, and it will load onto your computer. You must have Flash/Shockwave installed to view the animations. A link to a free download of Flash/Shockwave is provided online. While the animation is loading, you will see a loading status bar indicating the progress of the animation. When you are finished with the animation, close the window. Do not use the **Back** key, as the animation will remain open.

Video Clips

Approximately 180 video clips demonstrate how to perform key examination techniques and procedures. The links to the video clips are in each chapter folder, where appropriate. Click on the video you want to see. In some cases, there are several versions of the same examination. These are comparisons to show variation such as age or gender. The QuickTime Player must be installed to view the video clips. A link to a free download of the QuickTime Player is provided online. Three speeds of each video clip are available to view (56K, Cable/DSL, and CD), depending on your access capabilities. If you are using a dial-up connection (modem), you may want to use the *56K* link or the *CD-ROM* link. Accessing the video clips from the CD-ROM requires a simple installation. For instructions on running the installer on the CD-ROM, see page 13. Otherwise, you should use the *Cable/DSL* link. Loading the videos may take two or three minutes, especially if you are using a low-speed connection. While each video clip is loading, the QuickTime loading bar will show your progress.

Interactive Exercises

The interactive exercises are comprised of approximately 250 exercises for 28 chapters using 14 different online games. A description of each game is given below. Once you finish playing a game, your score will be displayed in the bottom left-hand corner of the window. There is no scoring report provided after you close the exercise. You may play the game as many times as you like, or you may stop in the middle of a game and start over. You must install Flash/Shockwave to access the exercises. A link to the free download of Flash/Shockwave is provided online. When you load each individual interactive exercise, a loading status bar appears.

- *Choose It*—Choose the answer that completes the sentence. You must identify the correct answer before you can move on to the next term. Correct answers are highlighted in blue. You can use the **Next** button after choosing the correct answer. Scoring is based on the first choice. Use the **Back** button to view previous questions. Reviewing questions does not change the score.

- *Flash Cards*—Choose a mode and click the **Begin** button to start. For each card, click the correct response. In Test Mode, each card appears once. You will not see your score until you have completed all cards. In Practice Mode, incorrect answers are shuffled back into the deck and will appear again. When you answer correctly, the card will be turned over. Scoring is based on the first attempt. Subsequent attempts are not penalized.

- *Hangman*—Click the lettered buttons to reveal the hidden word. If you choose the correct letter, it will appear in the blanks everywhere it occurs. For each incorrect answer, a part of the Hangman figure will appear. To win a game and score a point, reveal the hidden text before the Hangman is complete. You must complete each item before you can move on to the next term. Use the **Back** button to view previous questions. Reviewing questions does not change the score. Use the **Next** button to return to questions not yet answered.

- *Label It*—Label the image by typing the correct term into each box. Some terms may be more than one word. Incorrect characters will appear in red. Hit **Return** or **Enter** to indicate your answer is complete. Correct answers will be outlined in green and the cursor will move to the next term. For items to be scored, you need to enter them correctly the first time. Subsequent attempts are not counted. The word or phrase will appear after three incorrect attempts.

- *Listen and Select*—Click the **Play** button next to each item number to hear a word or a phrase pronounced out loud. A list of choices will appear. Click the choice that correctly expresses the word or phrase in the text with the correct spelling, punctuation, and capitalization. When you click the right word, it will be highlighted in blue and the word will appear in the blank next to the button. Scoring is based on the first attempt. Subsequent attempts are not penalized. You may listen to the sound as many times as you like by pressing the **Play** button.

- *Match It*—Click and drag the word part, word, or phrase to match the correct definitions. When you correctly place an item, it will remain beside the definition. If the answer is wrong, it bounces back to the word list. Scoring is based on the first attempt. One point is awarded for each item correctly placed on the first try. If you are wrong, you do not gain or lose points for trying again.

- *Memory Match*—Click the tiles to turn them over. Match pairs of tiles. The game counts how many times you turn over tiles. Try to clear the board with as few clicks as possible. Finishing in 30 clicks is good; 20 clicks is outstanding! Can you clear the board in under a minute?

- *Missing Letters*—Each word has a clue above it. Enter the correct letters into the empty boxes to complete the word or phrase. When a word is completed, click **OK**. If all the letters in the box are correct, most of the boxes will turn green. Some boxes will turn red (red letters are used to solve the mystery answer at the end). Use red letters to form the final word or phrase. Scoring is based on the first try. Subsequent attempts are not penalized.

- *Odd One Out*—According to the question or description, click the image or text that does not match. You must identify the correct answer before you can move on to the next term. Confirmation of the correct answer will appear. Use the **Next** button to advance to the next question. Scoring is based on the first choice. Use the **Back** button to view previous questions. Reviewing questions does not change the score.

- *Order It*—Drag the terms to the box to create the proper sequence. The position within the box where you drop a term does not matter as long as the term is in the right sequence. Sequencing begins with the first term placed correctly. When you place a term correctly, it remains in the box. An incorrect answer bounces back to the word list. Scores are based on the first attempt. Subsequent attempts do not affect your score.

- ***Picture It***—Click and drag the appropriate term to match its correct illustration. When the term is correctly placed, it will remain in the box. Incorrect answers will bounce back to the word list. Scoring is based on the first attempt. Subsequent attempts are not penalized.

- ***Quiz Show***—Answer the questions correctly to win the dollar amount associated with each question. Click a box on the game board to make the question appear. If the answer is correct on the first try, you win that amount, but if it is wrong, the amount is deducted from your winnings. After the first try, you don't gain or lose any money for trying again. Click the **Return** arrow to return to the game board.

- ***Think It Through***—Type the correct answer in the box. Some blanks contain more than one word. If the answer you typed is incorrect, it will appear in red letters. Hit **Return** or **Enter** to indicate your answer is complete. For items to be scored, you need to enter them correctly the first time. Subsequent attempts are not counted. The word or phrase will appear after three incorrect attempts.

- ***True or False***—For each statement, click on either **True** or **False**. You must click the correct answer before you can move on to the next question. Once the answer is highlighted in blue (indicating a correct answer) you may proceed to the next question by clicking on **Next**. You may use the **Back** button to review completed questions. Reviewing questions does not affect your score. Use the **Next** button to return to questions not yet answered. Scores are not retained and are based on the first attempt.

WebLinks

The WebLinks provide links to hundreds of websites that contain content relevant to the chapter material. The links are annotated, organized by chapter, and appear in the chapter folders for ease of use.

Audio Clips

The audio clips allow you to become familiar with important lung and heart sounds. Click on the sound you want to hear, and listen to it online! The audio clips are only included in Chapters 18 and 19 (the lung and heart chapters). You must have the QuickTime Player installed to listen to the audio clips. A link to a free download of the QuickTime Player is provided online.

Image Collection

The image collection contains more than 800 full-color images from the textbook that you can use to study or to enhance presentations. Chapter by chapter, you are able to preview image thumbnails or open full-size versions before downloading the image to your computer. Image downloads are handled via standard browser functionality. To download a full-size image, right-click on the image and select **Save Picture As . . .**. Name the file accordingly and save it to a location on your hard drive.

Anatomical References

Click on the **Anatomical References** link to view still shots from the video clips with anatomical overlays. The anatomical references provide you the opportunity to envision the inside of the body from the outside.

Practice Tests

Numerous questions are provided for each chapter so you can test yourself before and after studying each chapter. Each time you take a practice test, you are provided with different questions from a large pool of questions. The process for taking a test varies depending on the system (Evolve, Blackboard, WebCT, etc.) the course is hosted on. Your scores will vary depending on the points your instructor has assigned to the questions in the assessment as well. If you have any questions about taking tests or your scores, please ask your instructor.

Glossary

The glossary contains definitions of the key terms from the book. You can scroll through the terms or find them by clicking on the appropriate letter.

Laboratory and Diagnostic Tests

The laboratory and diagnostic tests are taken from *Mosby's Diagnostic and Laboratory Test Reference, Sixth Edition*, by Pagana and Pagana. Sixty-five tests are provided for your reference.

TECHNICAL REQUIREMENTS

To use an Evolve Online Course, you will need access to a computer that is connected to the Internet and equipped with web browser software that supports frames. For optimal performance, it is recommended that you have speakers and use a high-speed Internet connection. However, slower dial-up modems (56K minimum) are acceptable.

Screen Settings

For best results, the resolution of your computer monitor should be set at a minimum of 800 x 600. The number of colors displayed should be set to "thousands or higher" (High Color or 16 bit) or "millions of colors" (True Color or 24 bit). To set the resolution:

Windows
1. From the **Start** menu, select **Settings** and **Control Panel**.
2. Double-click on the **Display** icon.
3. Click on the **Settings** tab.
4. In the **Screen area** use the slider bar to select **800 by 600 pixels**.
5. In the **Colors** drop down menu, click on the arrow to show more settings.
6. Click on **High Color (16 bit)** or **True Color (24 bit)**.
7. Click on **Apply**.
8. Click on **OK**.
9. You may be asked to verify the setting changes. Click **Yes**.
10. You may be asked to restart your computer to accept the setting changes. Click **Yes**.

Macintosh
1. Select the **Monitors** control panel.
2. Select **800 x 600** (or similar) from the **Resolution** area.
3. Select **Thousands** or **Millions** from the **Color Depth** area.

Web Browsers

Supported web browsers include Microsoft Internet Explorer (IE) version 6.0 or higher, Netscape Navigator 7.1 or higher, and Mozilla 1.4 or higher.

If you use America Online (AOL) for Web access, you will need AOL version 4.0 or higher **and** one of the browsers listed above. Earlier versions of AOL and Internet Explorer will not run the course properly and you will have difficulty accessing many features.

For best results with AOL:
- Connect to the Internet using AOL version 4.0 or higher.
- Open a private chat within AOL. (This allows the AOL client to remain open, without asking if you wish to disconnect while minimized).
- Minimize AOL.
- Launch one of the recommended browsers.

Whichever browser you use, the browser preferences must be set to enable cookies as well as Java/JavaScript, and the cache must be set to reload every time.

Enable Cookies

Browser	Steps
Internet Explorer (IE) 6.0 or higher	1. Select **Tools**. 2. Select **Internet Options**. 3. Select **Privacy** tab. 4. Use the slider (slide down) to **Accept All Cookies**. 5. Click **OK**. -OR- 4. Click the **Advanced** button. 5. Click the check box next to **Override Automatic Cookie Handling**. 6. Click the **Accept** radio buttons under **First-party Cookies** and **Third-party Cookies**. 7. Click **OK**.
Netscape 7.1 or higher	1. Select **Edit**. 2. Select **Preferences**. 3. Select **Privacy & Security**. 4. Select **Cookies**. 5. Select **Enable All Cookies**.
Mozilla 1.4 or higher	1. Select **Tools**. 2. Select **Privacy**. 3. Expand the Cookies section and check the following box: Allow sites to set cookies.

Enable Java

Browser	Steps
Internet Explorer (IE) 6.0 or higher	1. Select **Tools -> Internet Options**. 2. Select **Advanced** tab. 3. Scroll down the list until you see the **Java (Sun)** section and select the box that appears below it.
Netscape 7.1 and higher	1. Select **Edit -> Preferences**. 2. Select **Advanced**. 3. Select **Scripts & Plugins**. 4. Make sure the **Navigator** box is checked to **Enable JavaScript**. 5. Click **OK**.
Mozilla 1.4 or higher	1. Select **Tools**. 2. Select **Web Features**. 3. Select the boxes next to **Enable Java** and **Enable Javascript**.

Set Cache to Always Reload a Page

Browser	Steps
Internet Explorer (IE) 6.0 or higher	1. Select **Tools -> Internet Options**. 2. Select **General** tab. 3. Go to the **Temporary Internet Files** and click the **Settings** button. 4. Select the radio button for **Every visit to the page** and click **OK** when complete.
Netscape 7.1 and higher	1. Select **Edit -> Preferences**. 2. Select **Advanced**. 3. Select **Cache**. 4. Select the **Every time I view the page** radio button. 5. Click **OK**.
Mozilla 1.4 or higher	1. Select **Tools**. 2. Select **Privacy**. 3. Expand the **Cache** section and designate a disk space number if one isn't in place already.

Plug-Ins

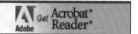

Adobe Acrobat Reader—With the free Acrobat Reader software you can view and print Adobe PDF files. Many Evolve products offer documents in this format, including student and instructor manuals, checklists, and more.

Download at: http://www.adobe.com

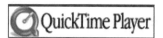

Apple QuickTime—Install this to hear word pronunciations, heart and lung sounds, and many other interesting audio clips within Evolve Online Courses.

Download at: http://www.apple.com

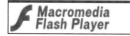

Macromedia Flash Player—This player will enhance your viewing of many Evolve web pages as well as educational short-form to long-form animation within the Evolve Learning System.

Download at: http://www.macromedia.com

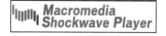

Macromedia Shockwave Player—Shockwave is best for viewing the many interactive learning activities within Evolve Online Courses.

Download at: http://www.macromedia.com

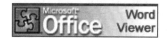

Microsoft Word Viewer—With this viewer, Microsoft Word users can share documents with others who don't have Word software. Users without Word can then open and view Word documents. Many Evolve products have test banks, student and instructor manuals, and other documents available for download and viewing on your local computer.

Download at: http://www.microsoft.com

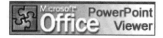

Microsoft PowerPoint Viewer—This viewer makes it possible for you to view PowerPoint presentations even if you don't have PowerPoint software. Many Evolve products have slides available for download and viewing on your local computer.

Download at: http://www.microsoft.com

LOGIN INSTRUCTIONS

IMPORTANT NOTE: These instructions apply only to users whose course is running on the Evolve Learning System. If you are taking an instructor-led course, please ask your instructor which system is hosting your course and where to find applicable instructions. Evolve courses can be run on a variety of systems and your instructor will decide which one is right for a particular course.

1. Go to: http://evolve.elsevier.com/student

2. Enter your username and password in the **Login to My Evolve** area and click the **Login** button.

3. You will be taken to your personalized **My Evolve** page where your course will be listed in the **My Courses** module.

SELF-ENROLLMENT INSTRUCTIONS

IMPORTANT NOTE: These instructions apply only to individuals who will be taking the course on their own. By taking the course independently, you will not have any instructor to help you with the course. You will have 12 months from the date you are enrolled to complete the course.

1. Go to: http://evolve.elsevier.com/Jarvis

2. Under the **Online Course** heading, click on the **Self-Study Student? Enroll Here** option. This will launch the enrollment wizard for your course.

3. Complete the enrollment wizard. During this process you will create an Evolve username and password. You will also be asked to provide identifying information about yourself and will need to provide the access code from inside the front cover of this guide.

4. Once the wizard has been completed you will be able to log in to your Evolve account and begin your Online Course immediately.

SUPPORT INFORMATION

Technical support is available to customers in the United States and Canada from 7:30 AM to 7:00 PM, Central Time, Monday—Friday by calling, toll-free: **1-800-401-9962**. You can also send an email to evolve-support@elsevier.com.

There is also **24/7 Support Information** available on the Evolve Portal (http://evolve.elsevier.com) including:

• Guided Tours
• Tutorials
• Frequently Asked Questions (FAQ)
• Online Copies of Course User Guides
• And much more!

VIDEO CD-ROM INSTALLER INSTRUCTIONS

Windows
1. Insert the CD-ROM.
2. Double-click on Setup.exe on the CD.
3. Follow the instructions on installer screens.
4. Restart your computer. You MUST restart your computer to complete the installation.

Macintosh
1. Insert the CD-ROM.
2. Double-click on the VPGSynch Installer icon.
3. Follow the instructions on installer screens.
4. Restart your computer. You MUST restart your computer to complete the installation.

Certain combinations of operating systems and Web browsers require additional set up to support the Video CD-ROM. Please refer to the "Read Me" section on the CD-ROM or the "Before You Begin" section of your course for additional instructions.

Video Clip Title

Video Clip Descriptor

Video Clip Title	Video Clip Descriptor
Inspection: Skin, Upper Extremities	Older Adult Male
Inspection: Skin, Back	Younger Adult Female
Inspection and Palpation: Pulses, Lower Extremities	Older Adult Female
Inspection: Nails of the Feet	Older Adult Female
Inspection and Percussion: Respirations and Diaphragmatic Excursion	Adult Male
Palpation: Lymph Nodes, Head, and Neck	Adult Male
Palpation: Upper Extremities and Lymph Nodes	Adult Male
Inspection: Face, Head, and Hair	Adult Male
Inspection: Face, Head, and Hair	Older Adult Female
Palpation: Face	Adult Male
Palpation: Face	Adult Female
Palpation: Face	Younger Adult Male
Palpation: Face	Younger Adult Female
Palpation: Face	Older Adult Male
Palpation: Face	Older Adult Female
Inspection: Neck	Younger Adult Female
Inspection: Neck	Older Adult Female
Inspection: Palpation and Range of Motion, Neck	Adult Male
Inspection: Palpation and Range of Motion, Neck	Older Adult Male
Inspection and Palpation: Carotid Pulse and Tracheal Alignment	Adult Male
Palpation: Thyroid (Anterior Approach)	Adult Male
Palpation: Thyroid (Anterior Approach)	Younger Adult Male
Palpation: Thyroid (Anterior Approach)	Younger Adult Female
Palpation: Thyroid (Posterior Approach)	Adult Male
Palpation: Thyroid (Posterior Approach)	Younger Adult Male
Inspection and Palpation: External Eye	Adult Male
Inspection and Palpation: External Eye	Adult Female
Inspection and Palpation: External Eye	Younger Adult Male
Inspection and Palpation: External Eye	Older Adult Male
Inspection and Palpation: External Eye	Older Adult Female
Inspection: Pupil Responses, Direct and Accommodation	Adult Male
Inspection: Eye Fixation Using the Cover-Uncover Test	Adult Male
Inspection: Six Cardinal Fields of Gaze	Adult Male
Inspection: Peripheral Fields of Vision	Adult Male
Inspection: Blink Reflex Using Corneal Sensitivity	Adult Male
Inspection: Red Light Reflex	Adult Male
Evaluation: Central Vision and Visual Acuity	Adult Male
Inspection: Eye Alignment	Older Adult Female
Inspection: Pupil Responses, Direct and Consensual	Older Adult Female

Evaluation: Hearing	Adult Male
Inspection: External Ear	Adult Male
Inspection and Palpation: External Ear	Adult Female
Inspection and Palpation: External Ear	Younger Adult Male
Inspection and Palpation: External Ear	Younger Adult Female
Inspection and Palpation: External Ear	Older Adult Male
Inspection and Palpation: External Ear	Older Adult Female
Inspection: Ear Canal	Adult Male
Hearing Evaluation: Rinne and Weber Tests	Adult Male
Hearing Evaluation: Rinne and Weber Tests	Older Adult Male
Hearing Evaluation: Rinne and Weber Tests	Older Adult Female
Inspection: Nose	Adult Male
Inspection: Nose	Adult Female
Inspection: Nose	Younger Adult Male
Inspection: Nose	Older Adult Male
Inspection: Nose	Older Adult Female
Evaluation: Smell	Adult Male
Inspection: Lips and Mouth	Adult Male
Inspection: Oropharynx, Teeth, and Tongue	Adult Male
Inspection: Oropharynx, Teeth, and Tongue	Older Adult Female
Inspection: Teeth	Adult Female
Inspection: Teeth	Older Adult Male
Evaluation: Gag Reflex	Adult Male
Evaluation: Taste	Adult Male
Inspection and Palpation: Breathing and Diaphragmatic Excursion, Anterior Chest	Adult Male
Inspection and Palpation: Respirations, Respiratory Excursion, and Tactile Fremitus, Posterior Chest	Adult Male
Palpation: Tactile Fremitus, Anterior Chest	Adult Male
Palpation: Tactile Fremitus, Posterior Chest	Adult Female
Inspection and Percussion: Diaphragmatic Excursion	Adult Male
Inspection and Percussion: Diaphragmatic Excursion	Younger Adult Male
Percussion: Anterior Thorax	Adult Male
Percussion: Posterior Thorax	Adult Male
Auscultation: Breath Sounds, Anterior Chest	Adult Male
Auscultation: Breath Sounds, Posterior Chest	Adult Male
Auscultation: Breath Sounds, Anterior Chest	Adult Female
Auscultation: Breath Sounds, Anterior Chest	Younger Adult Female
Inspection: Jugular Venous Distension	Adult Male
Inspection and Palpation: Cardiac, Anterior Chest	Adult Male
Inspection and Palpation: Cardiac, Anterior Chest	Adult Female
Inspection and Palpation: Cardiac Ausculatory Landmarks	Adult Male

Auscultation: Heart	Younger Adult Female
Auscultation: Cardiac, with Diaphragm	Adult Male
Auscultation: Cardiac, with Bell	Adult Male
Auscultation: Cardiac, with Diaphragm and Bell	Adult Female
Inspection: Capillary Refill, Upper Extremities	Adult Male
Inspection and Palpation: Upper Extremities and Pulses	Younger Adult Male
Palpation: Pulses and Lymph Nodes, Upper Extremities	Adult Male
Auscultation: Carotid Artery	Adult Male
Inspection and Palpation: Pulses, Lower Extremity	Adult Male
Inspection and Palpation: Pulses, Lower Extremity	Adult Female
Inspection and Palpation: Pulses, Lower Extremity	Older Adult Female
Inspection and Palpation: Pulses, Lower Extremity	Older Adult Female
Auscultation: Abdomen, Vascular Assessment	Adult Male
Palpation: Abdomen for Aortic Pulse	Adult Male
Inspection: Female Breasts (Sitting Position)	Adult Female
Inspection: Female Breasts (Sitting Position)	Younger Adult Female
Palpation: Female Breasts (Supine Position)	Adult Female
Palpation: Female Breasts (Supine Position)	Younger Adult Female
Palpation: Male Breasts (Supine Position)	Adult Male
Palpation: Male Breasts (Sitting Position)	Younger Adult Male
Inspection: Abdomen	Adult Male
Inspection: Abdomen	Adult Female
Inspection: Abdomen	Younger Adult Female
Inspection: Abdominal Wall Muscles	Adult Male
Inspection: Abdominal Wall Muscles	Younger Adult Male
Inspection: Abdominal Wall Muscles	Younger Adult Female
Auscultation: Abdomen, Bowel Sounds	Adult Male
Auscultation: Abdomen, Vascular Assessment	Adult Male
Percussion: Abdomen	Adult Male
Percussion: Liver	Adult Male
Percussion: Spleen	Adult Male
Palpation: Abdomen, Superficial and Deep	Adult Male
Palpation: Abdomen for Aortic Pulse	Adult Male
Palpation: Liver	Adult Male
Evaluation: Reflex, Abdominal Superficial	Younger Adult Male
Inspection: External Genitalia	Younger Adult Female
Inspection: Speculum Examination	Younger Adult Female
Palpation: Bimanual Examination	Younger Adult Female
Inspection and Palpation: Genitalia (Supine Position)	Younger Adult Male
Inspection and Palpation: Genitalia (Standing Position)	Younger Adult Male
Inspection and Palpation: Genitalia (Standing Position)	Younger Adult Male

Inspection and Palpation: Inguinal Hernia Evaluation	Younger Adult Male
Palpation: Inguinal Canal and Femoral Pulses (Supine Position)	Younger Adult Male
Palpation: Inguinal Canal and Femoral Pulses (Standing Position)	Younger Adult Male
Inspection: Buttocks and Anus	Younger Adult Male
Palpation: Rectal and Prostate Examination	Younger Adult Male
Inspection: Gait	Adult Male
Inspection: Gait	Older Adult Male
Inspection: Gait	Older Adult Female
Inspection: General Muscular Strength	Adult Male
Inspection and Palpation: Range of Motion, Neck	Adult Male
Inspection and Palpation: Range of Motion, Neck	Older Adult Male
Inspection and Palpation: Spine for Alignment	Adult Male
Inspection and Palpation: Spine for Alignment	Younger Adult Female
Palpation: Back	Older Adult Female
Inspection and Palpation: Upper Extremities and Capillary Refill	Adult Male
Inspection and Palpation: Upper Extremities and Pulses	Younger Adult Male
Inspection and Palpation: Range of Motion, Upper Extremities	Adult Male
Inspection and Palpation: Range of Motion, Upper Extremities	Younger Adult Male
Inspection and Palpation: Range of Motion, Upper Extremities	Older Male Adult
Inspection and Palpation: Range of Motion, Upper Extremities	Older Adult Female
Inspection and Palpation: Muscle Strength, Upper Extremities	Older Adult Male
Inspection and Palpation: Muscle Strength, Upper Extremities	Younger Adult Male
Inspection and Palpation: Range of Motion, Shoulders	Adult Male
Inspection and Palpation: Respirations and Diaphragmatic Excursion, Anterior Chest	Adult Male
Inspection and Palpation: Lower Extremities	Adult Male
Inspection and Palpation: Lower Extremities	Adult Female
Inspection and Palpation: Lower Extremities	Younger Adult Female
Inspection and Palpation: Lower Extremities	Older Adult Male
Inspection and Palpation: Lower Extremities	Older Adult Female
Inspection and Palpation: Pulses, Lower Extremities	Older Adult Female
Inspection and Palpation: Muscle Strength Evaluation, Lower Extremities	Adult Male
Inspection and Palpation: Muscle Strength Evaluation, Lower Extremities	Older Adult Male
Inspection and Palpation: Muscle Strength Evaluation, Lower Extremities	Older Adult Female
Inspection and Palpation: Range of Motion, Ankles and Feet	Adult Male
Inspection and Palpation: Range of Motion, Ankles and Feet	Older Adult Male
Inspection and Palpation: Range of Motion, Ankles and Feet	Older Adult Female
Inspection and Palpation: Stability and Range of Motion, Hips	Adult Male

Inspection: Cranial Nerves	Adult Male
Inspection: Cranial Nerves	Older Adult Female
Inspection: Fine Motor Coordination, Upper Extremities	Adult Male
Inspection: Fine Motor Coordination, Lower Extremities	Adult Male
Inspection: Fine Motor Coordination, Upper Extremities	Older Adult Male
Inspection: Fine Motor Coordination, Lower Extremities	Older Adult Female
Evaluation: Sensory, Face	Adult Male
Evaluation: Cremasteric Reflex	Younger Adult Male
Evaluation: Sensory, Upper and Lower Extremities	Adult Male
Evaluation: Sensory, Face and Upper Extremities	Older Adult Male
Evaluation: Sensory, Lower Extremities	Adult Female
Evaluation: Sensory, Light Touch; Face, Upper and Lower Extremities	Adult Male
Evaluation: Sensory, Light Touch; Face, Upper and Lower Extremities	Older Adult Male
Evaluation: Sensory, Face, Upper and Lower Extremities	Older Adult Female
Evaluation: Vibratory, Upper and Lower Extremities	Adult Male
Evaluation: Vibratory, Upper and Lower Extremities	Older Adult Male
Evaluation: Two-Point Discrimination	Adult Male
Evaluation: Two-Point Discrimination	Older Adult Male
Evaluation: Two-Point Discrimination	Older Adult Female
Evaluation: Stereognosis	Adult Male
Evaluation: Graphesthesia	Adult Male
Evaluation: Kinesthesia Movement	Adult Male
Evaluation: Deep Tendon Reflexes; Biceps, Triceps, and Brachioradialis Tendons	Adult Male
Evaluation: Deep Tendon Reflexes; Biceps, Triceps, and Brachioradialis Tendons	Adult Female
Evaluation: Deep Tendon Reflex, Patellar Tendon	Adult Male
Evaluation: Deep Tendon Reflex, Achilles Tendon	Adult Male
Inspection: Evaluation of Balance	Adult Male
Inspection: Evaluation of Balance	Older Adult Male
Inspection: Evaluation of Balance	Older Adult Female
Evaluation: Balance Using Romberg Test	Adult Male
Evaluation: Balance Using Romberg Test	Older Adult Male
Evaluation: Balance Using Romberg Test	Older Adult Female
Evaluation: Balance Using Heel-to-Toe Walking	Adult Male
Evaluation: Balance Using Heel-to-Toe Walking	Older Adult Male
Evaluation: Balance Using Heel-to-Toe Walking	Older Adult Female